The Essential Guide To Eating Paleo

The Stone Age Diet Revisited

By: Derrick Moore

TABLE OF CONTENTS

Publishers Notes 3

Dedication 4

Chapter 1- What Does It Mean To Eat Paleo? 5

Chapter 2- The Benefits of Eating Paleo 9

Chapter 3- What Are Some Meal Plans in the Paleo Diet? 13

Chapter 4- Is The Paleo Diet Healthy And Does It Help You To Lose Weight? 17

Chapter 5- 10 Paleo Breakfast Recipes 22

Chapter 6- 10 Paleo Lunch Recipes 29

Chapter 7- 10 Paleo Dinner Recipes 35

About The Author 44

PUBLISHERS NOTES

Disclaimer

This publication is intended to provide helpful and informative material. It is not intended to diagnose, treat, cure, or prevent any health problem or condition, nor is intended to replace the advice of a physician. No action should be taken solely on the contents of this book. Always consult your physician or qualified health-care professional on any matters regarding your health and before adopting any suggestions in this book or drawing inferences from it.

The author and publisher specifically disclaim all responsibility for any liability, loss or risk, personal or otherwise, which is incurred as a consequence, directly or indirectly, from the use or application of any contents of this book.

Any and all product names referenced within this book are the trademarks of their respective owners. None of these owners have sponsored, authorized, endorsed, or approved this book.

Always read all information provided by the manufacturers' product labels before using their products. The author and publisher are not responsible for claims made by manufacturers.

© 2013

Manufactured in the United States of America

DEDICATION

This book is dedicated to my parents.

CHAPTER 1- WHAT DOES IT MEAN TO EAT PALEO?

Just imagine yourself consuming a daily diet plan of fruits, vegetables, lean meat and seafood. With the Paleo diet your carb intake is derived purely from the veggies and natural fruits, and you would also have load of fiber in your diet. Your food will be low on sodium and sugar, but there will be ample potassium. Actually, this is the diet that our ancestors followed millions of years ago. The amount of nutrients our ancestors ate is a far cry in comparison to what we consume today.

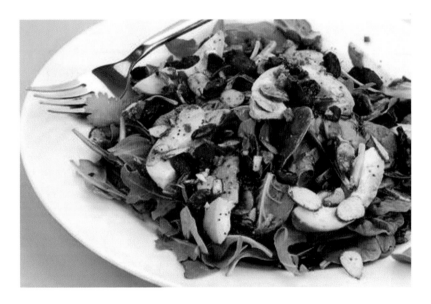

There has been a very little evolution in the past 14,000 years. Therefore, we've been genetically programmed to eat pretty different from what we actually eat today. Our dietary habits have changed dramatically. There is also a shift in the disease patterns from the health issues due to the nutrient deficiencies and the infectious problems to chronic degenerative diseases due to the unbalanced and excessive intake of nutrients and energy. In Paleolithic age, the leading cause of fatalities used to be various infectious diseases, but these days it is because of various degenerative disorders due to the excessive or unbalanced intake of vitamins and minerals.

The Paleo diet is considered to be the best diet which is based largely on the lean meat and food items that promote longevity and health. Our Paleolithic ancestors never consumed baked beans or granola bars. In the past 14,000 years only few of our genes have changed and our biological machinery is still the same. The processed foods and refined carbohydrates, added sugars, and vegetable oils in the modern treats are a high glycemic load that raises blood sugar levels and also burdens insulin production, which promotes atherosclerosis and inflammation.

Even though early humans consumed more than 3,000 calories a day, intense physical activity kept the weight gain at a minimum. Our very existence indicates that diets our ancestors ate provided them with sufficient nutrients and energy to support growth and reproduction. Today with highly processed and abundant food supply and minimal work expenditure required to obtain it, most of the people end up consuming excess calories resulting in unwanted fat.

Is Paleo Diet Easily Available?

Thankfully everything you need to follow the Paleo diet is easily available. The biggest benefit of Paleo diet is the complete removal of refined and processed foods from your diet. Paleo diet focuses on maximizing the amount of protein in the diet. This protein is obtained from the nuts, veggies, fruits, unprocessed grains and lean meat. In fact, research suggests that scavenged nuts and fish provided far more energy than pizzas or hotdogs you eat today. Oil fresh fish in a Paleo diet is much better than cuts from the mammals that are stacked with unhealthy fats.

You should also include fruits, dairy vegetables, grains and lean meats, healthy fats and avoid processed food, sugars, seafood, legumes, nuts & seeds, starches, and alcohol in your Paleo diet. Another rich protein source that can be used in the Paleo diet is eggs that are from organically fed, free range chickens. The ones you gather from your own back yard chicken coop would be the best ever, as this food source is free from hormones, antibiotics and other contaminants!

The best thing about Paleo diet is that it is low on sodium and sugar and is high in proteins, which provided the optimum health to our ancestors that lived in the Paleolithic era. While Paleo diet's main priority is health, it is also good for weight loss. All those who developed this diet believe that cave man that existed in the Paleolithic era had the healthiest diet that helped him live a disease free life and provided sufficient energy without adding unwanted fat to the body.

During the Stone Age, there was no need for the processed or instant foods with a longer shelf life. It was only in the last few decades that fast and convenient preparations have been introduced in the market to make life easier for the busy people. All these items contain preservatives and chemicals and are not good for our health. These are the reasons why the Paleo diet has gained widespread popularity.

Health Benefits of the Paleo Diet

When you shift to a Paleo diet, you will see increased weight loss, improved blood lipids, and reduced inflammation and pain the body. However, many people are not inclined to blindly follow all the recommendations, whether they are related to the exercises or nutrition. Some folks want to know why they are doing something different. Fortunately, the Paleo diet has successfully stood the test of time, and the rigors of the scientific scrutiny. With a simple shift you can easily remove all food that are at odds with your health and can also increase your mineral, vitamin and antioxidant intake.

Can You Afford It?

Many people want to know whether Paleo diet recipes are more expensive than the "normal food". Well, some people think that staying on a Paleo diet would bankrupt them, but the reality is that Paleo diet is not at all expensive. In fact, it is much cheaper than the processed foods that are available on the market. Aside from that, there are so many Paleo diet recipes available online that will make your switch from the normal diet to the Paleo diet the most painless one.

Best of all, a person on Paleo diet will be able to use the food to the maximum and nothing will be thrown away any longer. There will be no need for refrigeration in the moldy fridges and this diet is best for all those who are on a budget. If you really end up with lots of fruit and vegetables left over, you can simply make a smoothie. If lot of meat is left over, you can simply turn it into a Paleo soup or a stew. So, with a Paleo diet, there is no way you will be stuck with tons of leftovers making it extremely healthy and cost effective at the same time.

Chapter 2- The Benefits of Eating Paleo

The Paleo Diet, which is also known as the Caveman Diet, is one of the more unique concepts to emerge in health and fitness circles. It would be difficult to call it a new diet since it is based on eating habits that first emerged during the era of the caveman. Yes, this is a diet based on how people ate during the Paleolithic Era, an era that ended over 10,000 years ago but began several million years prior to that.

The obvious fact about the diet is that many of the modern problems associated with processed food did not exist during the Paleo era. While many excellent and progressive innovations have emerged regarding the way food is produced and stored, there have been quite a number of drawbacks that emerged health wise. Through the rediscovery of the Paleo Diet, a host of those annoying dietary problems based on a poor modern diet can be addressed.

The Core of the Paleo Diet

At the core of the Paleo Diet would be the eating of very simple food choices. Meats and seafood, fruits and vegetables, and nuts are the core staples. Refined sugars, grains, dairy, and anything processed are absolutely not part of the diet whatsoever. Basically, if our ancestors did not eat it, then the selection is not going to be part of the Paleo Diet.

A common question will arise here among those who are not Paleo fanatics. Basically, why do this? What are the benefits of the Paleo Diet?

On the surface, it might seem like this diet is yet another in a long line of fads. That is not the case at all. There are quite a number of very positive benefits to eating Paleo. Those willing to take the time out to try the Paleo Diet and stick with it for an extended period of time might quickly learn the diet can offer a host of improvement beyond mere weight loss.

The Weight Loss Factor

Even those it was just mentioned to look beyond the basic benefit of weight loss, the truth is the potential to lose a lot of weight is possible. The food selections in the Paleo Diet are generally low in calories. The obvious exception would be red meat due to the high fat content in certain selections. (Those opting to eat red meat are well advised to select the leaner cuts of meat) The bulk of the selections in the Paleo Diet are also low in carbohydrates with fruit being the notable exception. The sugars in fruit are, of course, natural. As a result, they have much less of a negative impact than the refined sugars found in processed food choices.

Most people feel the need to go on a diet because they want to lose weight. There is certainly nothing wrong with this desire. The common problem many have with so many diet plans is it is never easy to find a diet that actually works and can yield the desired results. The Paleo Diet is definitely one capable of contributing to weight loss. The low calorie and low sugar amount makes not losing weight difficult.

There are other benefits to eating Paleo and these benefits have contributed strongly to the popularity of the diet.

The Somewhat Overlooked Additional Benefits of Eating Paleo

Improvements in overall health would be among the top benefits of eating selections from the Paleo Diet. The fats found in this diet are commonly referred to as the good fats thanks to the positive effects they have on the cells and even on the brain. Omega three fatty acids are found in a number of the food selections and these fats can greatly aid in improving heart health quite a bit.

Chapter 3- What Are Some Meal Plans in the Paleo Diet?

The Paleo Diet is often referred to as the Cave Man diet or the Stone Age diet. It is a modernized plan that is based on the ancient diet of our ancestors which was usually made up of wild plants and animals. It includes meal plans that are made up of domesticated animal meat and cultivated plants. These are all foods that can be hunted, planted or fished such as seafood, eggs, fruit, nuts, vegetables, meat, mushrooms, herbs and seeds.

Many individuals who would like to lose weight and maintain a healthy lifestyle are interested in starting the Paleo diet. This diet plan does not require any additional supplements or high-priced meal deliveries. Instead a person simply has to alter their eating habits and take on a more natural approach when it comes choosing food to eat. Choosing to start on a Paleo diet plan can help an individual to lose weight, gain more energy, and take part in more physical activities than ever before. Here are a few helpful meal plan ideas that anyone can use to get started on the popular Paleo Diet.

Paleo Diet Meal Plans for Breakfast

For individuals on the Paleo diet, breakfast can include a variety of favorites such as eggs, bacon and fresh fruit. Breakfast may be the most important meal of the day, but it does not have to be the largest. Prepare two to three slices of bacon with a side of two eggs fixed however you prefer. You can also choose to drink your breakfast by creating a Green Smoothie using Kale and Kiwi. A bowl of fresh strawberries and bananas can make a refreshing morning meal, and for something a little different, you may want to try sausage with sautéed broccoli sprouts or Paleo pancakes served with blueberries or strawberries.

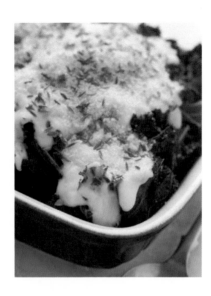

Lunch Ideas for Those on the Paleo Diet

For lunch, there are many options for individuals on the Paleo diet plan. Enjoy a large salad made with romaine lettuce or grilled chicken strips with steamed asparagus. A serving of cooked mixed vegetables with strip steak can be a healthy meal choice and tuna salad served with apple slices is an easy idea for lunch to take along with you to school or work. You may also want to try simple meals such as a hamburger patty with cooked spinach, steamed vegetables with grilled chicken, or pork chops served with sweet potatoes.

Dinner Meal Plans for the Paleo Diet

Dinner is usually the largest meal that those on the Paleo diet eat. Some of the most popular dinner meal plans include Bison burger patty with steamed vegetables, Grilled shrimp salad served with a romaine lettuce and spinach salad, Salmon and avocado, grilled stead with mashed cauliflower, rotisserie chicken with sliced apples, Grilled tuna with celery, and Grilled chicken served with a side of mixed berries.

Beverage Ideas for the Paleo Diet

Paleo dieters have the advantage of trying out a variety of festive beverages for everyday dinners or holiday meals. Try out a warm pumpkin latte for upcoming fall events or a fun pumpkin spice latte. The Christmas cranberry cocktail made with pink grapefruits, vodka and liquid Stevia is an extra special drink, and the World's Best Sangria is a delicious beverage to enjoy during the warm summer months.

Paleo Desserts

While most of our favorite desserts are loaded with sugar, there are some Paleo-friendly options out there that can help take care of everyone's sweet tooth. Fresh fruit without any added sugar is always an option and can be eaten alone or mixed into a delicious smoothie. For some extra special treats, try grilled bananas, grilled peaches, or dip your favorite fruits into a sweet Paleo-friendly fruit dip. All-natural banana ice cream can be made by blending bananas and placing the creamy concoction into the freezer overnight.

A festive fall treat that uses Paleo-approved ingredients is Pumpkin Brownies. These snacks can be prepared for Halloween, Thanksgiving or for any fall dinner. To make these delicious brownies, you will need Coconut cream concentrate, eggs, raw organic honey, pumpkin puree, organic cocoa powder, cinnamon, pumpkin pie spice, vanilla extract, baking soda and sea salt. Top the brownies with homemade pumpkin frosting made with vegetable shortening made with palm oil, raw organic honey, vanilla and pumpkin pie spice.

Holiday Meal Ideas for the Paleo Lifestyle

The holidays can be a difficult time for anyone on a diet. But it is possible to still have a Thanksgiving feast or Christmas dinner while sticking to your Paleo diet plan. The turkey can be prepared using four tablespoons of grass fed organic butter, and seasoned with stalks of rosemary and thyme. Appetizers can include Crab Stuffed Mushrooms prepared with minced chives, dried thyme, roasted red peppers and dried oregano, and Prosciutto Wrapped Pears prepared with thinly

15

sliced red onion, prosciutto di parma, baby spinach leaves, coconut oil and balsamic vinegar. For side dishes, go with traditional stuffing mixed with Italian pork or chicken sausage and seasoned with garlic powder, celery and yellow onion. Paleo Holiday Yams include fresh grated ginger, ground cinnamon and 100% pure maple syrup.

While Thanksgiving is probably the biggest holiday of the year when it comes to preparing delicious food, you will also need to come up with tasty dishes for many other special occasions. Some Paleo-inspired recipes you may want to try for the holidays or a special family dinner are Saffron Salmon, Smokey Turkey Chili, Apple Omelets, Garlic Basil Chicken Spaghetti, Slow-Cooked Barbeque Pork Loin and Paleo Beef Stew prepared in the slow cooker.

How to Find Out More about Paleo Diet Meal Plans

There are many online blogs and websites that are dedicated to explaining how to live the Paleo lifestyle. These helpful sites and blogs feature unique recipes for Paleo-style entrees that you can easily prepare at home. If you are planning on switching to the Paleo diet and would like to find out more information on how this simple diet plan can change your entire life, you should check out one or more of these exceptional websites, Everyday Paleo, Ultimate Paleo Guide and Paleo Diet Lifestyle.

CHAPTER 4- IS THE PALEO DIET HEALTHY AND DOES IT HELP YOU TO LOSE WEIGHT?

The Paleo diet is healthy and can help you lose weight. In general, the Paleo diet has been tested by nutritionists and found to be as healthier than the Mediterranean diet, diabetes prevention diets, and the normal diet that most people in the United States and other western countries consume.

The healthfulness of the Paleo diet has been studied since 2007 and confirmed to be safe and healthy in several small studies and meta-reviews by experts in nutrition and health from leading universities in the United States and in Europe.

The Paleo diet has been found to be superior to most western diets and to Mediterranean diets in producing weight loss. This effect has been confirmed in clinical studies reported in major medical publications in the United States and Europe.

Like most diets, one should not expect miracle weight loss from the Paleo diet. You can expect to drop as much as five pounds in three weeks with the Paleo diet with no exercise. Some studies have reported women that lost as much as 75 pounds in six months by following the Paleo diet rigorously.

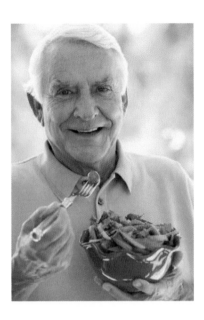

You can improve weight loss by adding an exercise routine to the Paleo diet. The Paleo diet does not actively support any particular exercise routines.

You can improve your weight loss by making calorie conscious choices with the Paleo diet. One of the ways to avoid calories is to avoid fat in meat. The Paleo diet is a carnivore diet so picking meat with lower fat means lower calorie intake and more weight loss.

One thing the Paleo diet offers for weight watchers and dieters that is superior to other diets is no calorie counting. The food content of the Paleo diet makes calorie counting and any record keeping unnecessary.

You do not have to give up sweets with the Paleo diet. The Paleo diet provides sweets in the form of fruit, a variety of plants, mushrooms, and truffles.

The Paleo diet is basically a very low carbohydrate (low carb) diet. This fact benefits your weight loss strategy and can also help prevent type 2 diabetes. Type 2 diabetes is self-induced by eating too much and eating refined sugars, large amounts of carbs, sweets, and dairy products. The

Paleo diet eliminates refined sugars, minimizes carbs, and cuts out sweets and dairy products. The Paleo diet can prevent type II diabetes but cannot prevent type 1 diabetes but the Paleo diet can help manage type 1 diabetes because the intake of carbohydrates is reduced. Carbohydrates are the big problem in diabetes.

The Paleo diet recommends consuming about ten percent more fat than is recommend by the Food and Drug Administration of the United Sates and the National Institutes of Health. You have options with the Paleo diet so weight loss goals can be achieved and heart health concerns can be addressed by eating less fat and leaner meats.

Some studies have shown that the Paleo diet reduces blood pressure, LDL cholesterol (the bad kind) and triglycerides.

The Paleo diet provides 50 percent of the FDA recommendation for carbohydrates for adults. The energy need from the carbs you would eat is provided by meat and fruit. Low carbs help with weight loss and can help prevent type 2 diabetes from developing.

The Paleo diet exceeds recommended protein requirements by 11 to 20 percent depending on your sex and how big you are. The added protein is an energy source and with exercise can turn fat into muscle and provide added weight loss.

The Paleo diet is very low salt. Low salt is particularly important for people that have kidney disease, high blood pressure, and diabetes.

The Paleo diet is high fiber from all the fruit and vegetables. Fiber improves digestion and regularity. The sugar from fruit is processed differently than sucrose so you do not gain weight. The fruit and vegetables also provide a huge variety of vitamins. Antioxidants in fruit are a free radical scavenger that is known to help prevent cancer.

The Paleo diet provides almost twice the amount of potassium than the FDA recommends. Potassium is necessary for the sodium potassium pump to produce proper nerve function. Potassium also helps prevent kidney stones and reduces bone loss. Most people do not get enough potassium in their diet.

The Paleo diet provides more B-12 vitamins than are recommended by the FDA. Most people do not get the recommended amount of B-12 vitamins. B-12 vitamins are critical in mitochondrial energy production and cell metabolism.

The Paleo diet is not a perfect food source. The normal person using the Paleo diet will not get the FDA recommended amounts of calcium or vitamin D. The solution to the problem is supplements. Calcium and Vitamin D are recommended as supplements to the Paleo diet. Thirty minutes of sunlight exposure is needed three times a week to convert vitamin D into a useable form even if you are not using the Paleo diet.

If you do not like fish or shell fish the Paleo diet recommends the use of omega-3 fish oils as a supplement to provide the fatty acids that are in fish.

One of the most productive factors in the Paleo diet for weight loss is the feeling of fullness that eating meat and fruit produces. The feeling of satiation (fullness) produces a cascade of chemical reactions in the brain that tell you are full. The onset of this chemical process can produce feelings of fullness that last for hours. This helps you lose weight because you do not experience cravings or the afternoon munchies.

The low glycemic index foods in the Paleo diet prevent spikes in blood glucose. This is important for people that are diabetic in maintaining the right sugar balance. This fact also helps people maintain weight loss by preventing cravings that go along with glucose spikes and drops.

The Paleo diet can produce substantial weight loss and can help keep weight under control if followed rigorously.

Like all diets the Paleo diet has some drawbacks that prevent it from being the diet for everyone. If you chose the Paleo diet you should be aware of the nutritional requirements the diet does not provide and make a routine of using supplements (calcium and vitamin D) to provide what the Paleo diet does not.

The Paleo diet is healthy for most people who do not have a physical condition that requires a special diet.

CHAPTER 5- 10 PALEO BREAKFAST RECIPES

One of the most popular lifestyle diets is known as the Paleo Diet. It is centered on the notion of eating like the "cavemen" did during ancient times. More commonly illustrated, however, is the concept of hunters and gatherers. Foods like plants, berries, and natural meat are game; consequently, candies, pastas, and processed foods are off limits. Below you will find 10 of the most popular Paleo breakfast recipes.

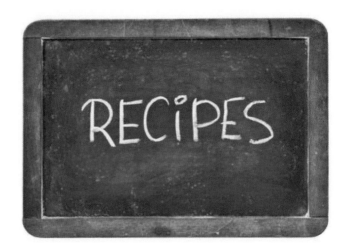

Western Omelet

Ingredients

4 eggs
1/2 diced onion
1/4 lb. Of ham
1 bell pepper, chopped
1 teaspoon of coconut oil
1 medium tomato, diced
1 cup of spinach

Sea salt and pepper

Directions

Chop the vegetables, and crack and beat the eggs into a bowl. Heat skillet over medium heat, and add the coconut oil. Next, pour half of the eggs into the skillet, allow sitting, and then add half of the vegetables and ham. When they have settled in, flip one half of the egg over the ham and vegetables, allow to sit for 2 minutes, and enjoy.

Banana Carrot Muffins

Ingredients

2 cups of almond flour
2 teaspoon of baking soda
1 teaspoon of sea salt
1 tablespoon of cinnamon
3 eggs
1 cup of dates
3 bananas (ripe)
1 teaspoon of apple cider vinegar
1/4 cup of coconut oil
1 1/2 cup of carrots
3/4 cup of walnuts

Directions

Preheat the oven to 350 degrees Fahrenheit. Combine the cinnamon, sea salt, baking soda and flour. In a food processor, mix the eggs, bananas, dates, apple cider vinegar, and coconut oil. Add the liquid mixture to the dry mixture and fold in nuts and carrots. Spoon mixture onto a sheet and bake for 25 minutes.

Bacon Stir-Fry

Ingredients

8 bacon slices
1/2 onion, diced
1 sweet potato, diced
1 zucchini, diced
8 green beans
1 avocado

Directions

Chop and cook the bacon in a skillet over high heat (drain the fat when done). Heat another pan over medium heat and add 1 tablespoon of dripping from the bacon pan, onion, and sweet potato and sauté for about 15 minutes. Then add the green beans and zucchini to the potato mixture. Combine the bacon and vegetables and enjoy.

Almond Flour Pancakes

Ingredients

1 cup of almond flour
1/2 cup of applesauce (unsweetened)
2 eggs
1/4 cup of water
1 tablespoon of coconut flour
1/4 teaspoon of sea salt
1/4 teaspoon of nutmeg
Coconut oil
Berries

Directions

Add the flour, applesauce, eggs, nutmeg, water, and sea salt into a container and mix thoroughly. Add 1 teaspoon of coconut oil to a medium heated frying pan. Add 1/4 cup of batter into the pan, and flip it like a normal pancake. Top with fresh berries and repeat.

BLT Breakfast

Ingredients

6 bacon slices
2 cups of spinach
1 cup tomatoes (cherry)
4 eggs
1 avocado
2 tablespoons of almonds

Directions

Cook the bacon in a big, medium heated skillet for about fifteen minutes. Set aside 1 tablespoon of the bacon drippings, then add the tomatoes and baby spinach to the bacon. When the tomatoes and spinach are warm, remove them from the heat. Next, heat another pan over medium flame, and add the bacon drippings that you had set aside, and fry the eggs in it. When finished, serve and enjoy.

Smoked Salmon Scrambled Eggs

Ingredients

1 teaspoon of coconut oil
4 eggs
4 oz. smoked salmon
1 tablespoon of water
4 chives
1/2 avocado

Directions

Heat a skillet over medium flame, and add the coconut oil. Crack the eggs in a bowl, put in the water, and scramble. Then, add the eggs and salmon to the skillet. When finished, remove from heat and top with avocado, pepper and chives.

Steak and Eggs

Ingredients

1/2 lb. boneless beef steak
1/4 teaspoon of pepper
2 teaspoon of coconut oil
1 red bell pepper
1/4 teaspoon of sea salt
1/4 diced onion
Spinach
4 mushrooms
2 eggs

Directions

Heat a big pan over medium flame, and add 1 teaspoon of coconut oil, mushrooms, onions, and steak. Sauté until the steak is cooked. Add the spinach and pepper and cook. Heat another small frying pan, and add the rest of the coconut oil, and fry the eggs. Serve and enjoy.

Pumpkin Muffins

Ingredients

3/4 cup pumpkin
3 eggs
1 teaspoon of baking powder
1 1/2 cups flour (almond)
1 teaspoon of baking soda
1 1/2 teaspoon of pie spice (pumpkin)

1/2 teaspoon of cinnamon
1/4 cup honey
1/8 teaspoon of salt
2 teaspoons of almond butter
1 tablespoon of almonds

Directions

Preheat oven to three hundred and fifty degrees Fahrenheit. Coat the muffin tins with the coconut oil and mix all of the ingredients to pour into the tins evenly. Bake for twenty five minutes and sprinkle almonds on top after removing them from the oven.

Breakfast Smoothie

Ingredients

2 cups of berries
2/3 cup of shredded coconut
1 cup of almond milk
2 eggs

Directions

Place the frozen berries in a blender and add splashes of hot water. Next, add the coconut, eggs, and almond milk. Blend until smooth and then serve.

Tapioca Crepes

Ingredients

1 cup of tapioca flour
1 cup of canned coconut milk
1 egg
Sea salt

Toppings of your choice

Directions

Combine all of the ingredients into a bowl. Heat a skillet on medium heat, and pour 1/3 cup of mixture into the skillet. Cook both sides for about 2 to 3 minutes. Add your toppings and enjoy.

CHAPTER 6- 10 PALEO LUNCH RECIPES

The Paleo Diet is a diet oriented around working with your genetics to establish learner and stronger health. In essence, if you can't find it in nature, than you can't eat in. The diet uses the efforts of ancient gathering and consuming methods to receive proven results (so if candy and pasta is your thing, you might want to write a farewell speech).

The Paleo Diet offers a tremendous amount of benefits. It stabilizes blood sugar, burns off stored fat, improves sleep patterns, clears away skin oils and naturally strengthens your teeth. It also enhances your workouts, reduces allergies, and provides balanced energy throughout the day. Below you will find 10 popular lunch recipes that are sure to thrill your taste buds.

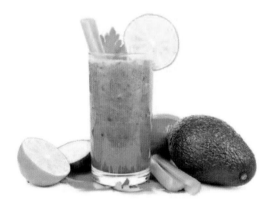

Green Smoothie

Ingredients

1 apple
1 pear
1/2 tablespoon of chopped ginger
2 tablespoons of flax seed
2 handfuls of spinach

Juice from 1 lemon
1 cup water

Directions

Remove the stems of the apple and pear, and put them into the blender. Then add the remaining ingredients and blend at a high level. Add more variations of vegetables and fruits to your liking.

Bone Broth

Ingredients

2 ibs of chicken bones
1 yellow onion, chopped
4 cups of vegetables
2 bay leaves
1 tablespoon of black peppercorns
1 tablespoon of oregano
1 tablespoon of funnel seed
1 teaspoon of thyme
1 tablespoon of sea salt
2 tablespoons of apple cider vinegar
Water

Directions

First, preheat the oven 350 degrees Fahrenheit. Spread the bones onto a sheet and roast for 20 minutes. Add the bones and the other ingredients to a large soup pot then cover the lid, and let simmer for 8 to 23 hours. Skim every few hours. Season with sea salt and consume within 24 hours.

Balsamic Asparagus Salad

Ingredients

1 ib. of asparagus
1 tablespoon of red onion, minced
1 tablespoon of extra virgin olive oil
4 teaspoons balsamic vinegar
1 clove minced garlic
Ground black pepper

Directions

Boil a medium pot of water. Add the asparagus and allow it to boil for 3 minutes. Drain, rinse, and dry the asparagus. Mix all other ingredients together and serve at room temperature.

Cilantro Turkey Burgers

Ingredients

1 cup chopped cilantro
1 lb. turkey (ground)
1/4 red onion, diced
2 teaspoon garlic
1 teaspoon sea salt
1/4 teaspoon black pepper

Directions

Place ingredients in a bowl and mix to combine then use a fork to blend. Divide the mixture into four portions and then make patties. Grill and serve.

Thai Chicken Wraps

Ingredients

12 roman lettuce leaves
1 ib. boneless chicken breasts

4 chopped cabbage leaves
1 cup chopped raw broccoli
3 onions (green)
1/4 cup of water
Cilantro
1/4 cup almond butter
2 tablespoons of coconut aminos
Juice of a lime
2 garlic cloves

Directions

Grill and dice the chicken breasts into 1/2 inch cubes. Spread the leaves out, and fill them with the chicken, broccoli, and other ingredients. Drizzle the Thai sauce and enjoy.

Sloppy Joes

Ingredients

2 tablespoons of coconut oil
1 onion, chopped
1 green pepper, chopped
2 cloves garlic, minced
1 lb. ground beef
1 can tomato sauce
1 tablespoon chili powder
1/2 teaspoon of ground cumin

Directions

Heat a large skillet on medium and add the oil and then sauté the onion, pepper, and garlic. Add the beef and cook for about 10 minutes. Finally, stir in the tomato sauce, chili sauce, and cumin.

Paleo Pizza

Ingredients

1 cup almond flour
2 beaten eggs
3 tablespoons of almond butter
1/2 teaspoon sea salt
3 teaspoons of olive oil
4 mushrooms
1/2 cup of diced onion
1 large sausage (Italian)
1 red pepper
2 cloves of garlic
1/2 cup of marinara sauce
1/2 teaspoon of dried oregano
1/2 cup of grape tomatoes

Directions

Preheat oven to 350 degrees Fahrenheit. Combine the sea salt, eggs, almond butter and almond flour. With two tablespoons olive oil, spread the mixture over a baking sheet then bake it for ten minutes. While this is baking, add the rest of the sliced sausage, mushrooms onions and oil to a heated skillet, and let cook for 4 to 6 minutes. Put the red pepper and garlic in the skillet. Take the crust out of the oven and cover it with marinara sauce, put in the vegetables, and bake for 25-30 minutes.

Spaghetti

Ingredients

1 tablespoon olive oil
2 cloves of garlic, chopped
1 lb. ground beef
15 oz. marinara sauce
24 oz. kelp noodles

Directions

Heat a large skillet on medium and add oil. Add meat and garlic. Add the noodles and sauce and let simmer.

Spicy Tuna Salad

Ingredients

2 cans of tuna
1 cup of black olives
2 chopped green onions
1 jalapeno pepper
3 tablespoons of caper
1/2 teaspoon of chili flakes
Juice of 2 lemons
Olive oil
1 avocado

Directions

Combine all of the ingredients and serve over lettuce. Enjoy!

Paleo PB&J

1 cup of berries
4 tablespoons of almond butter

Directions

Mix the berries and almond butter into a bowl and spread across a bread of your choice.

Chapter 7- 10 Paleo Dinner Recipes

Spicy Paleo Pulled Pork

Ingredients

Dry Spices

2/3 tbsp salt
1/3 tbsp paprika
1/3 tbsp dry mustard
1/3 tbsp cayenne pepper
2/3 tbsp chili powder

Meat

2-3 lb shoulder pork roast
1/8 cup of water
Sauce Ingredients
½ cup apple cider vinegar
1/3 cup spicy yellow mustard
2 ounces tomato paste
1 minced garlic clove
Pinch of salt
1/3 tsp cayenne pepper
1/6 tsp black pepper

Directions

Add all dry spice ingredients to a bowl and mix thoroughly

Thoroughly spread the dry rub mix over the entire cut of pork

Add pork and 1/8 cup of water to a crock pot; cook on medium-high for 6-7 hours

While pork is cooking, add all sauce ingredients to a pan; simmer in medium-low heat for 8-10 mins; set aside when finished

Drain cooked pork liquid into a bottomed pan and simmer for 10-15 mins; add to the sauce and cook for 5 mins

Use forks to carefully pull pork meat until stripped into shreds

Pour ½ of sauce onto shredded pork and set the other half aside for a dip

Serve as desired

Japanese Paleo Short Ribs

Ingredients

Meat

2 lbs beef short ribs
Spices
1/3 tbsp oil
1/3 chopped onion
2 garlic cloves
1 small hot pepper
2/3 tbsp fresh ginger root
1/3 cup beef stock
2/3 cup water
1/6 cup tamari soy sauce
1/12 cup white vinegar
2/3 tbsp fish sauce
2 ounces shitake mushrooms
1 -2 thinly sliced scallions
Pinch of salt
Pinch of pepper

Directions

Lightly season the beef ribs with salt and pepper

Add the ribs to an oven ready pan and sear on a stove for 1-2 mins, using medium-high heat. Set the beef aside and cover with foil. Sauté the chopped onion in the oven ready pan for ten mins

Add garlic, pepper and ginger to the pan and sauté for 1 minute; stir occasionally. Add the ribs and the rest of the ingredients to the pan

Bring the entire mix to a simmer, place in preheated 300 degree F oven for 3 hours. Remove the pan from the oven and remove ribs

Bring the sauce to a low boil and simmer for 15-20 mins

Add the shitake mushrooms and continue simmering for 5-8 mins

Return the beef to the pan and let cool for 5-10 mins and serve as desired

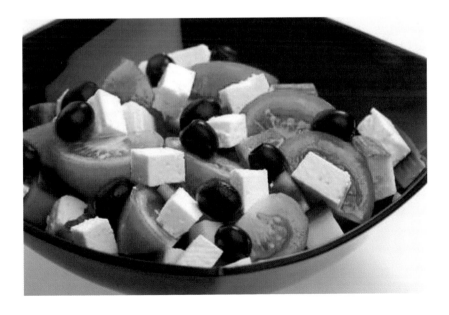

Chipotle Duck Breast

Ingredients

Meat

1 lb boneless duck breast
Pinch of salt
Pinch of pepper
Sauce
1 cup orange juice
Tbsp lime juice
1/4 tbsp finely chopped chipotle pepper
1 clove
1/3 tsp salt

Directions

Simmer all of the sauce ingredients in a saucepan using medium heat for 18-22 minutes; set aside

Carefully score the duck meat's skin and fat; sprinkle the duck with salt and pepper and sear over medium heat for 8 mins on each side

Pour half of the sauce onto the meat and set the rest aside for dipping

Serve as desired

Kale Salad and Beef Sausage Dressing

Ingredients

1/3 bunch kale
1 ounce diced beef sausage
¼ cup sliced mushrooms
¼ cup diced onion

2 tbsp olive oil
1 tbsp apple cider vinegar
Pinch of salt
Pinch of pepper

Directions

Sauté the sausage in a pan over medium heat using 1 tbspn of olive oil for 5 mins and add the mushrooms and onions to the pan and sauté for another 5 mins

Reduce the heat to low and add remainder of olive oil, vinegar, salt and pepper; simmer for 3 mins then tear the kale leaves into preferred size and add to a mixing bowl

Pour sauce over kale and serve as desired

Spicy Curry Squash and Avocado

Ingredients

1 tbsp red curry paste
1 minced clove garlic
1 minced chili pepper
1 cup chicken stock
1/3 tbsp fish sauce
½ can coconut milk
2 cups squash
1/3 lb boneless, skinless chicken breast
1 tbsp coconut oil
1 diced mushroom
1 avocado

Directions

Fry the curry paste, chili and garlic over coconut oil in a medium pot for 5 mins then add the chicken stock, coconut milk and fish sauce; bring to a low boil; reduce heat to low

Add the squash and simmer for 5-7 mins and add the chicken breast and simmer for another 5-7 mins

Add the mushrooms and simmer for 5 more mins and remove the pan from the heat and add avocado

Serve as desired

Tangy Alaskan Salmon

Ingredients

¾ lb Alaskan salmon
1 tbsp oil
1 tbsp lemon juice
Salt
Pepper
1/3 tbsp minced dill

Directions

Spread the oil in a baking pan and sprinkle the salmon with salt and pepper and add it to the pan

Mix the lemon juice and dill, and spread it over the salmon and add the pan to a preheated oven at 400 degrees F; bake for 10-12 mins

Let the salmon cool for 10 mins then serve as desired

Handmade Spicy Pork Sausages

Ingredients

½ lb ground pork
½ tsp dried sage
¼ tsp thyme
Pinch of salt
Pinch of pepper
¼ tbsp garlic powder
¼ tbsp coconut sugar
Pinch of red pepper flakes
½ tsp fennel

Directions

Add all ingredients to a mixing bowl; hand mix thoroughly

Make 3-6 patties with the mixture

Cook the patties over medium for 6 mins on each side

Place the cooked patties in an absorbent napkin, let cool for 5 mins and serve as desired

Late Night Curry Bacon Omelets

Ingredients

3 large eggs
3 strips of bacon
½ tbsp oil
Pinch of salt
Pinch of pepper
1/8 tsp curry powder
¼ minced onion

Directions

Add the bacon to a baking sheet; bake in preheated oven at 415 degrees F for 15-20 mins then add the oil to a preheated pan and mix all remaining ingredients in a mixing bowl

Add the mixing bowl ingredients to the pan; place bacon on top of the ingredients after 30 seconds

After 1 min, carefully fold the mixture over top of itself

After an additional min, flip contents of pan and cook for 1 min

Serve as desired

Chicken Salad over Kale

Ingredients

Meat
1 cup diced chicken
Salad Mix
½ cup diced sweet pepper
1 diced artichoke heart
2 thinly sliced scallions
1 large kale leaf
Pinch of parsley
¼ cup of avocado oil mayonnaise

Directions

Sauté the chicken until cooked thoroughly and add all ingredients, including chicken, to mixing bowl; thoroughly hand or spoon mix

Place the kale leaf on a plate and then spread the mixture over the kale leaf and serve as desired

Black Pepper Shrimp

Ingredients

¾ lb peeled shrimp
½ tbsp garlic powder
½ tbsp fish sauce
2/3 tbsp black pepper
Pinch of salt

Directions

Add the coconut oil to a preheated pan over medium heat and place the shrimp in a mixing bowl.

Mix the remaining ingredients in a separate mixing bowl; pour over the shrimp then pour the entire contents of the shrimp mixing bowl into the pan and sauté for 5 mins then serve.

ABOUT THE AUTHOR

Derrick Moore does not consider eating the Paleo way as a diet. For him, it is the only way to eat. It's healthy, natural, balanced, and has been around for a long time. We are the ones in the twenty first century now realizing what it's really about. He knows that nowadays, there are more health-conscience individuals than ever; as he is one himself. But Paleo really resonated with him to the point where he views it as an obligation to society to put a handy guide out on it.

This makes it a simple way for people to get educated about it or to be informed on how beneficial it really is for everyone. After seeing how pleased he is with eating the Paleo way, many of his family members have joined him in that direction. His wife, Rita, does not prepare meals any other way for their family. He feels this is the best way to eat and everyone should check it out and start eating this way too.